AF890186

Scan the QR code
to read and listen to the
glossary words for FREE!

glossary - Meanings of words.

Published in the UK by Every Cherry Publishing Limited, 2026
Unit 4u18, The Book Brothers Business Park, Tolwell Road,
Leicester LE4 1BR, United Kingdom

Every Cherry Publishing Limited
Unit 31, The Pottery, Bakers Point,
Pottery Road, Dún Laoghaire,
Dublin A96 EV18, Ireland

EVERY CHERRY and associated logos
are trademarks and/or registered trademarks of
Every Cherry Publishing Limited.

2 4 6 8 10 9 7 5 3 1

ISBN: 978-1-80263-704-5

Sherlock Holmes: A Study in Scarlet
Easier Classics

Adapted Text © Every Cherry Publishing Limited 2026
Illustrations © Sweet Cherry Publishing Limited 2019

Based on the original story by Sir Arthur Conan Doyle
Text adapted by Gemma Barder
Illustrations by Arianna Bellucci

All rights reserved. No part of this publication may be reproduced or utilised in any form or by any means, electronic or mechanical, including photocopying, recording, or using any information storage and retrieval system, without prior permission in writing from the publisher. No part of this publication may be used or reproduced in any manner for the purpose of training artificial intelligence technologies or systems.

www.everycherry.com

Printed and bound in Turkey

FSC
www.fsc.org
MIX
Paper | Supporting responsible forestry
FSC® C221129

Every Cherry

SHERLOCK HOLMES

A STUDY IN SCARLET

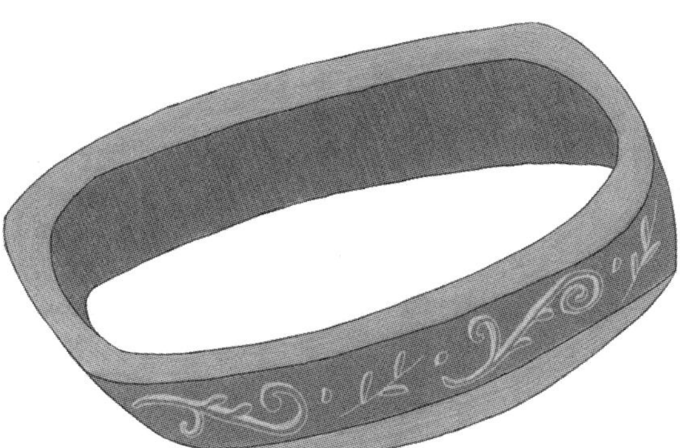

Meet the Characters

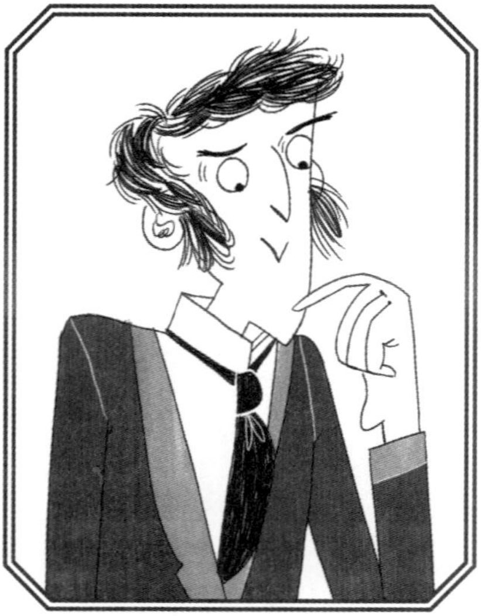

Sherlock Holmes

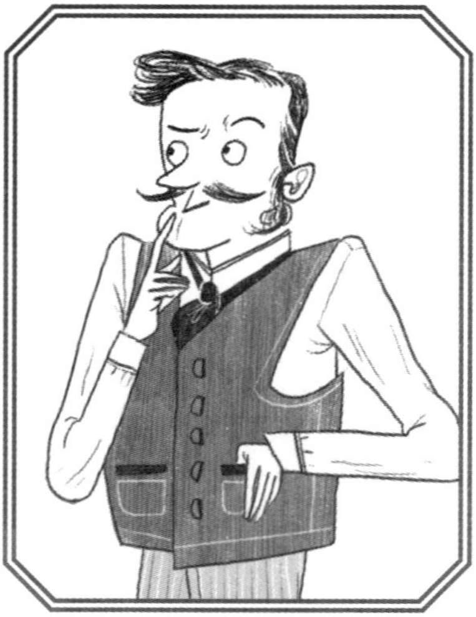

Doctor Watson

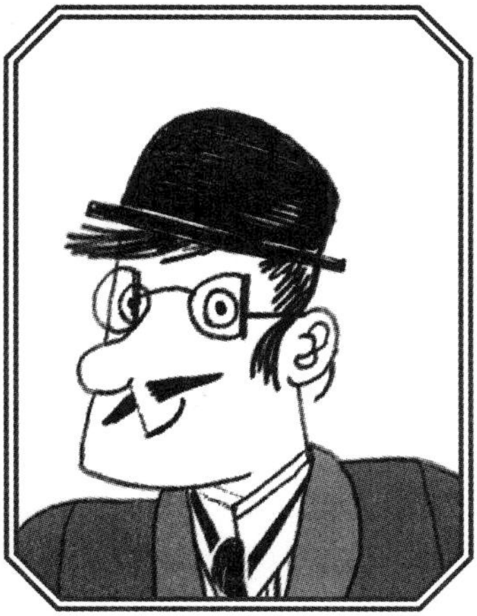

Stamford

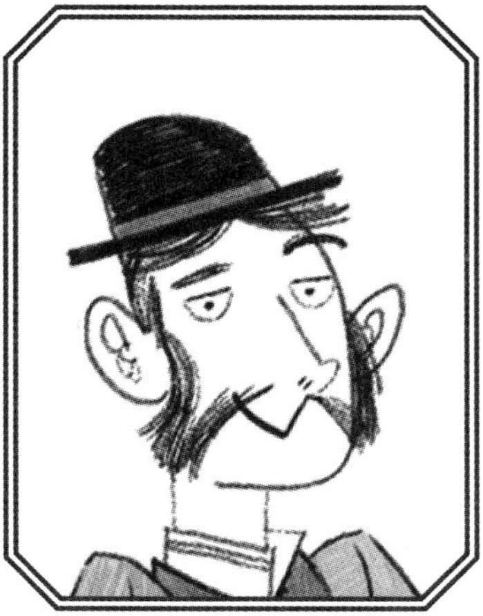

Detective Lestrade

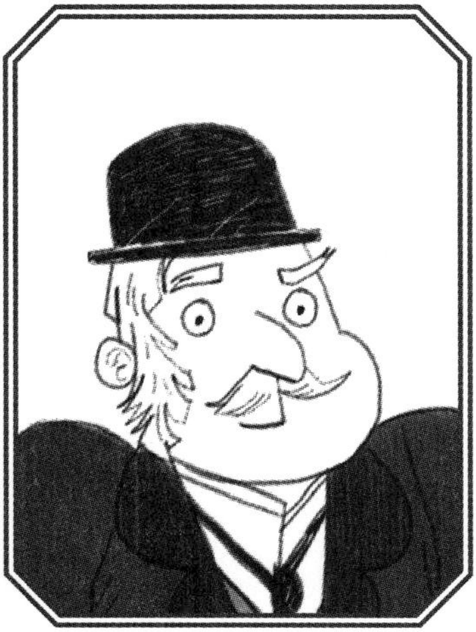

Detective Gregson

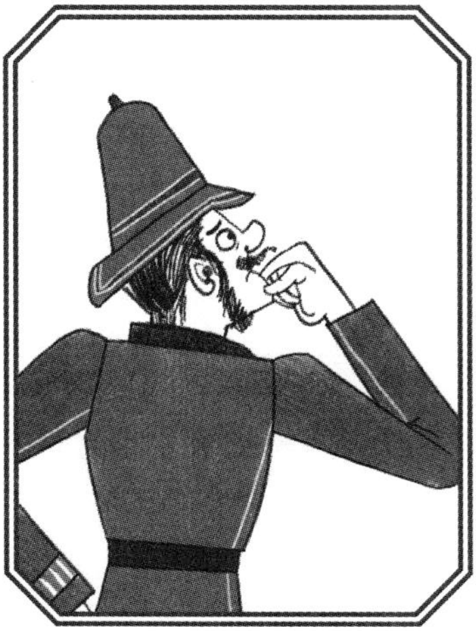

Constable Rance

Chapter 1

My name is Doctor Watson.

I used to be an ***army doctor*** *in* ***Afghanistan****, but I was* ***injured****. I could not work anymore, so I came back to London.*

I had nowhere to stay and only a small amount of money.

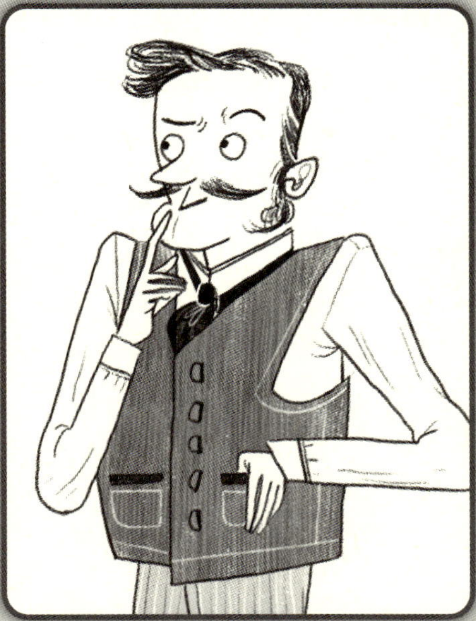

army doctor - A doctor who gives medical help to soldiers.

Afghanistan - A country in Asia.

injured - When part of the body has been hurt.

At first, I stayed in a hotel. The hotel was very nice but it cost too much money.

I met an old friend called Stamford at the hotel.

I told Stamford that I needed somewhere else to stay.

'I know someone else who is looking for a place to live too,' said Stamford. 'His name is Sherlock Holmes.'

'Can you **introduce** us?' I asked. 'Maybe we could find somewhere to live together.'

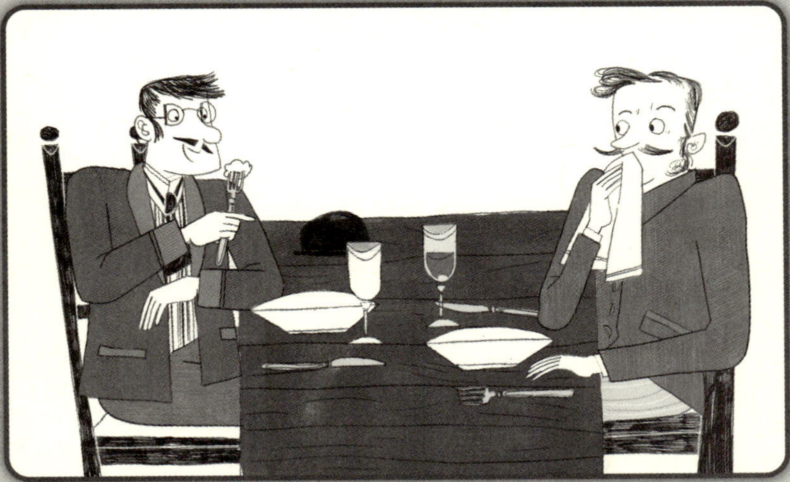

introduce - To tell two people each other's names so they can get to know each other.

Stamford frowned. 'I will introduce you,' he said. 'But I must tell you, Sherlock is an odd man.'

I was not worried. Some people think I am odd too. I still wanted to meet Sherlock.

We got into a **hansom cab**. It took us to see him.

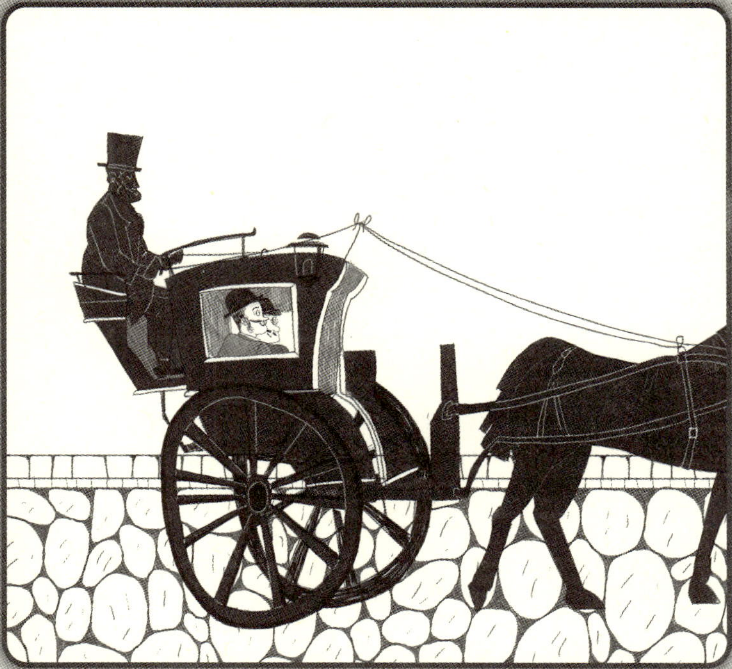

hansom cab – A Victorian carriage that is pulled by a horse and driven by a person. (A carriage is something people travel in.)

Chapter 2

Sherlock was working in a ***laboratory*** *at a hospital. Stamford introduced us.*

'Sherlock, this is Doctor Watson. He is looking for somewhere to live, just like you.'

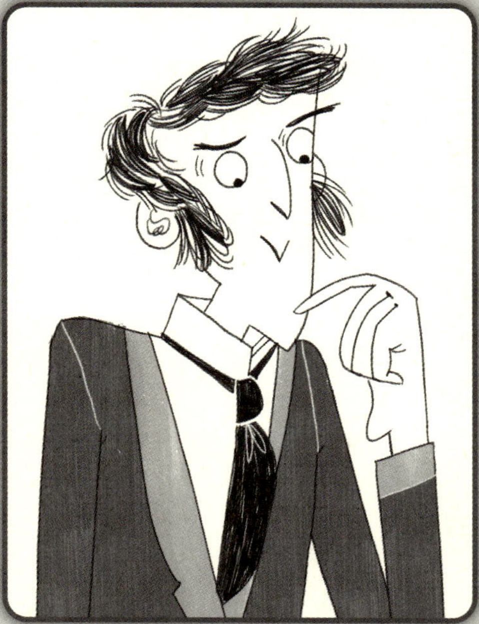

laboratory - A special room where scientific tests are done.

Sherlock shook my hand. 'It is good to meet you,' he said. 'You have just come back from Afghanistan, haven't you?'

I was shocked that he already knew this.

'How did you know?' I asked.

Sherlock laughed. 'Never mind! I will tell you later,' he said.

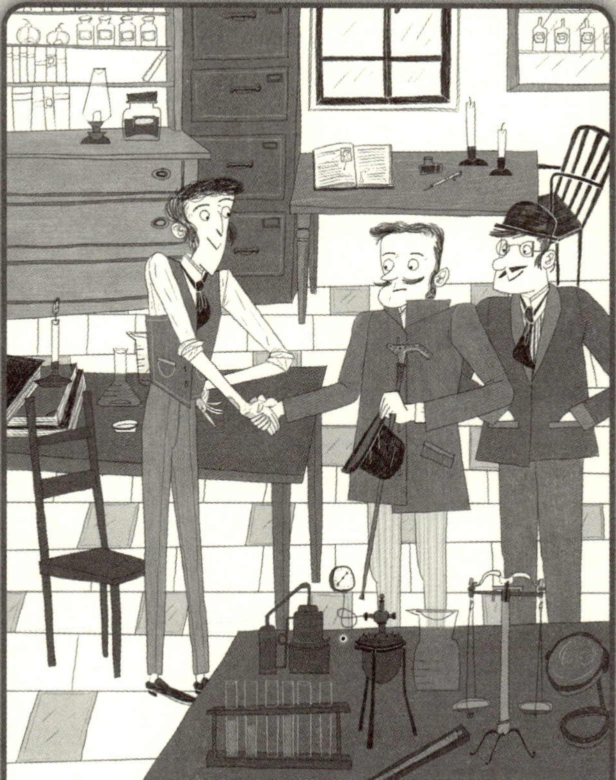

Sherlock had some questions to ask me before we agreed to live together.

'I **conduct experiments** at home sometimes,' he said. 'Would that worry you?'

'Of course not,' I replied.

'I also play the violin,' said Sherlock. 'Would that bother you?'

'Not at all!' I replied.

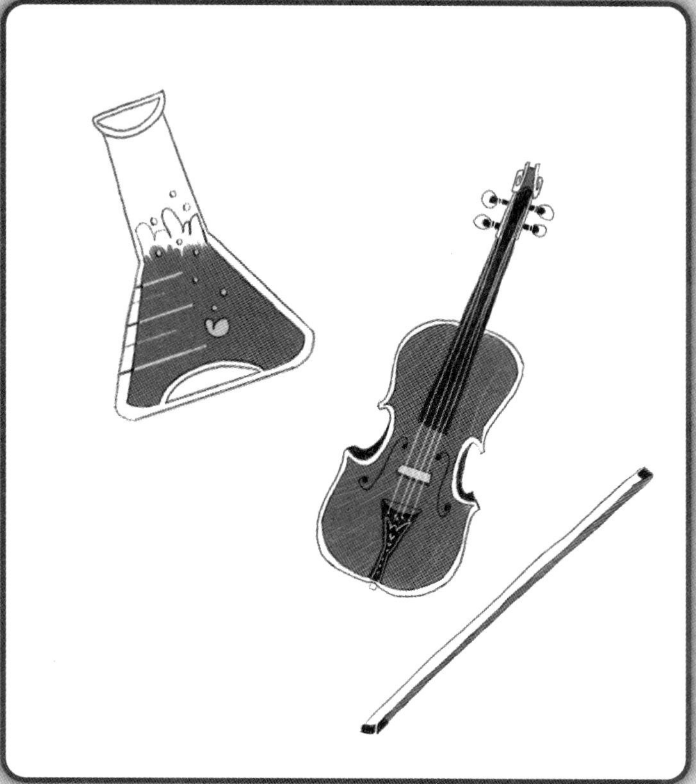

conduct - To carry out or do.

experiments - Scientific tests which are done in order to find something out.

Finally, I had a question for Sherlock.

'What is your job?' I asked.

Sherlock smiled. 'I ***solve mysteries*** *and* ***crimes****,' he said.*

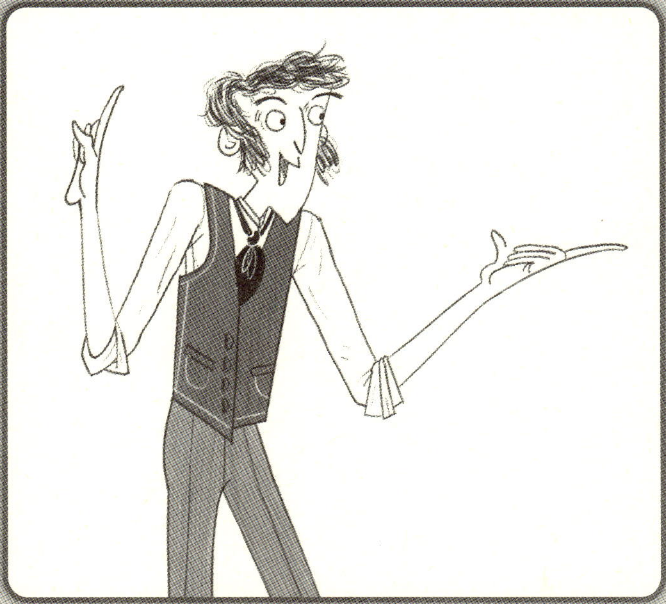

solve - *Find the answer to something.*

mysteries - *Events or things that are difficult to explain.*

crimes - *Actions or activities that break the rules of a country.*

Chapter 3

I was excited to move in with Sherlock. We lived in Flat 221B on Baker Street. It was a lovely place.

There was a kind **landlady**.
She cooked and cleaned for us.

landlady - A woman who allows people to live in a house she owns, in return for money.

I started to find out more about Sherlock. He knew lots about **science** and the **law**, but he was not interested in **politics**.

'I only like to learn things that are useful,' said Sherlock. 'Otherwise, my brain would be too full!'

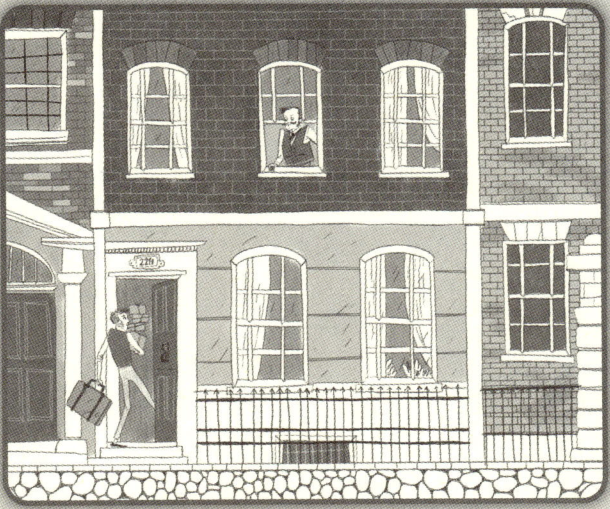

science - *Conducting experiments to discover more about the world.*

law - *A group of rules a country makes that people have to follow.*

politics - *The way in which a government runs a country.*

Sherlock spent some of his days working hard.

On other days he did nothing except sit on the sofa, looking sad.

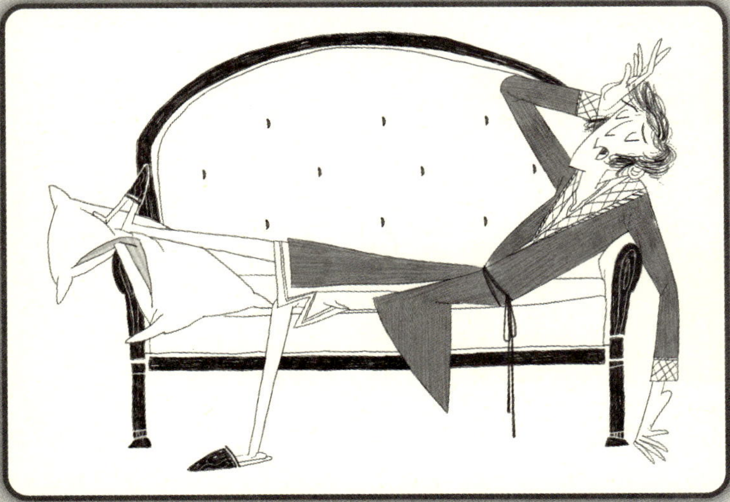

Sherlock had lots of visitors. Most of them wanted him to help them solve mysteries.

Sometimes Sherlock was visited by two ***detectives****. Their names were Detective Gregson and Detective Lestrade.*

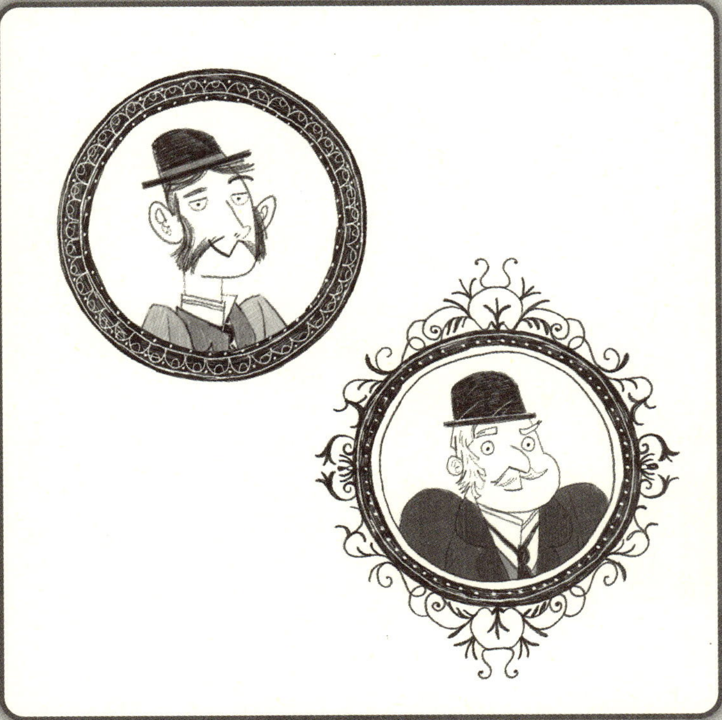

detectives - *People whose job is to discover what has happened in a crime and to find the people involved.*

Chapter 4

One morning, I asked Sherlock how he had known that I was an army doctor in Afghanistan.

'I knew the moment I saw you!' said Sherlock. 'Shall I explain?'

'Yes please,' I said.

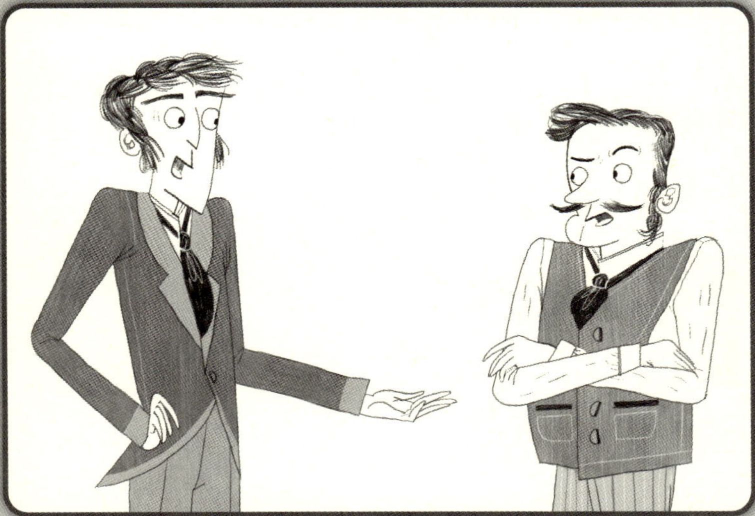

'You are calm and kind, just like a doctor,' said Sherlock. 'And you walk straight and tall, just like a soldier.'

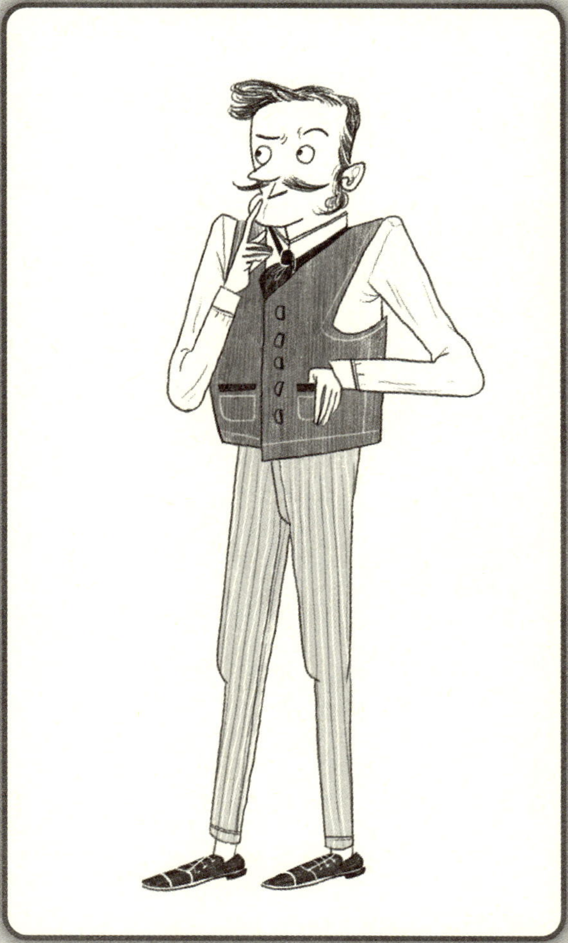

Next, he had seen that my arm was injured and my skin was **tanned**.

'So I knew that the army must have sent you home, probably from somewhere hot, like Afghanistan,' he said.

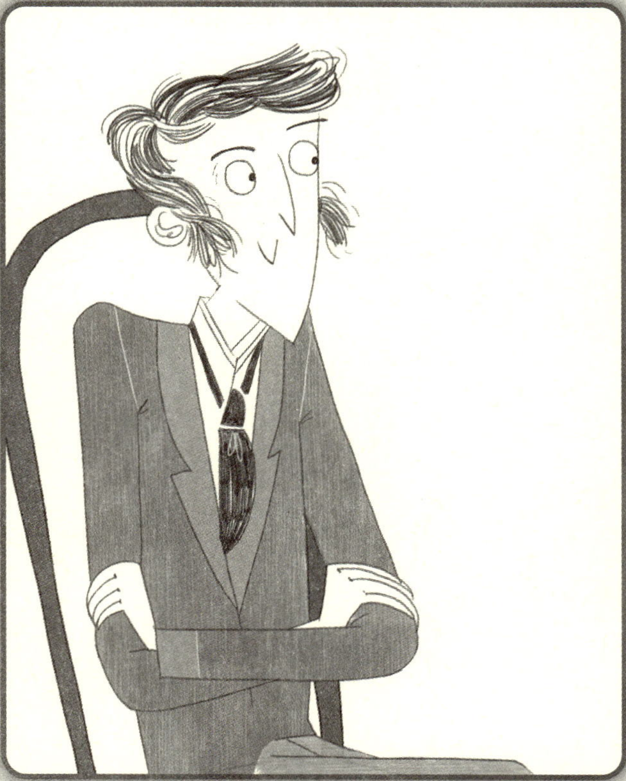

tanned - When skin has gone darker in the sun.

I stared at Sherlock in shock. I could not believe that he had known all of that just by looking at me.

Just then, a note was posted under our door. It was from Lestrade and Gregson, the detectives.

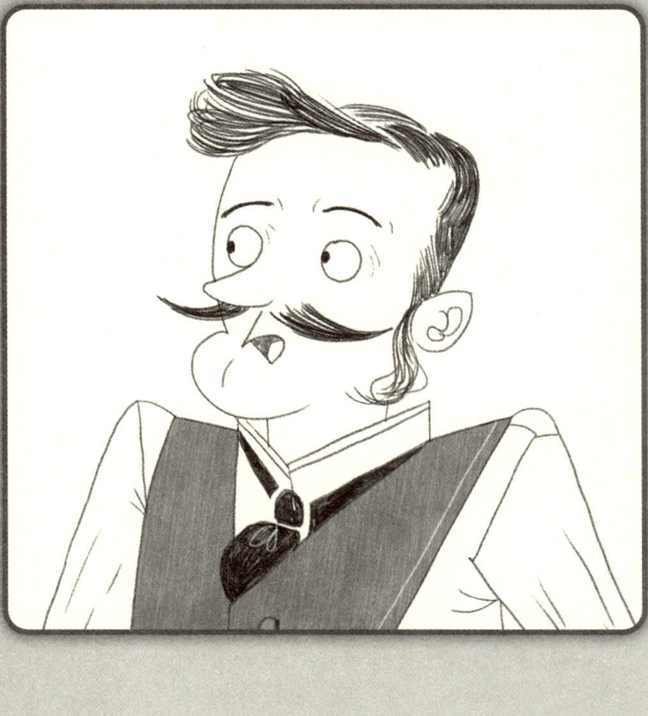

Chapter 5

The note asked Sherlock to meet the detectives straight away.

> **Please come to**
> **3 Lauriston Gardens.**
> **A body has been found.**
> **It looks like murder!**

Sherlock called for a hansom cab.

He asked me to go with him.

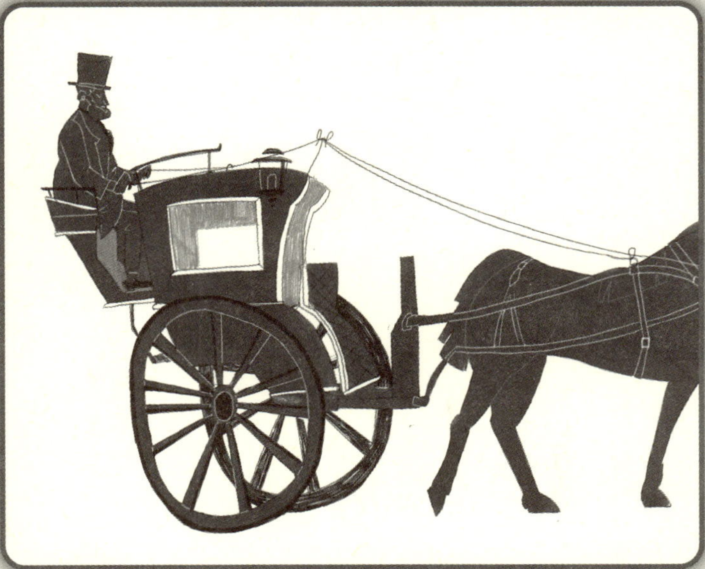

murder - When someone has been killed on purpose.

The hansom cab stopped a few streets away from Lauriston Gardens. Sherlock wanted to walk the rest of the way.

'I will look for **clues** on the way,' he said.

I walked beside him. I saw nothing, but Sherlock wrote lots of information in his notepad.

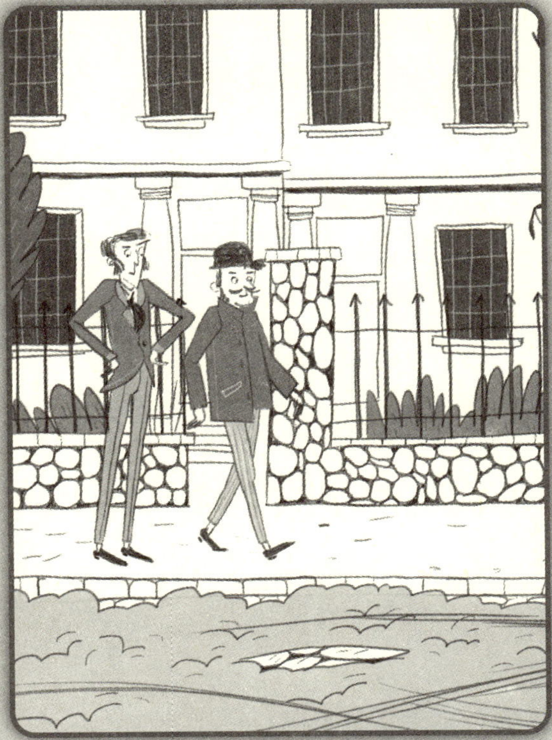

clues - *Pieces of information that help you find an answer or solve a crime.*

Gregson was waiting for Sherlock in the house.

'Thank you for coming, Sherlock,' said Gregson. 'Early this morning, a policeman found the body of a man.'

Sherlock walked slowly into the front room. 'This is a very serious crime,' he said.

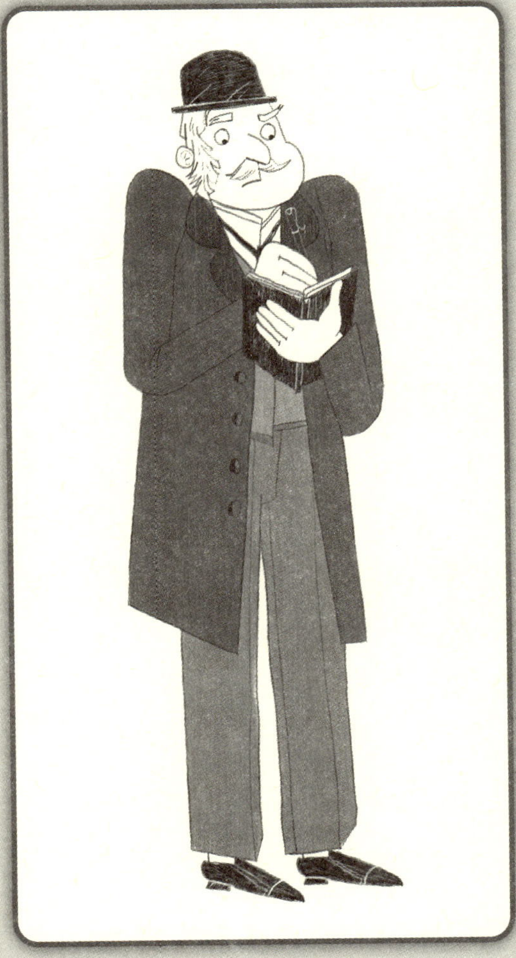

The front room was dirty and dusty. There was a single red candle in the corner.

The body of a man lay on the floor.

The body was dressed in smart clothes. A **top hat** lay next to it.

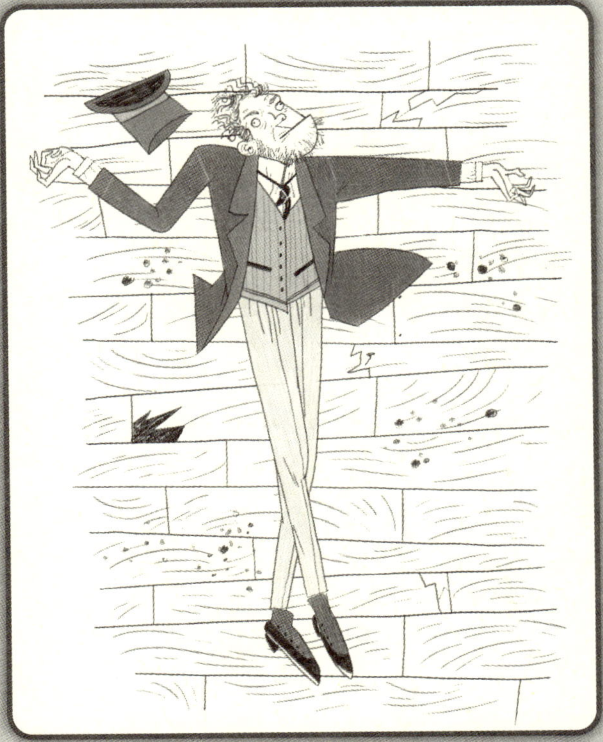

top hat - An old-fashioned hat, which is tall and narrow.

Chapter 6

Lestrade entered the front room.

'Are there any clues about how the man died?' he asked.

'No,' said Gregson, 'none at all.'

At that moment, Sherlock began to **inspect** the body.

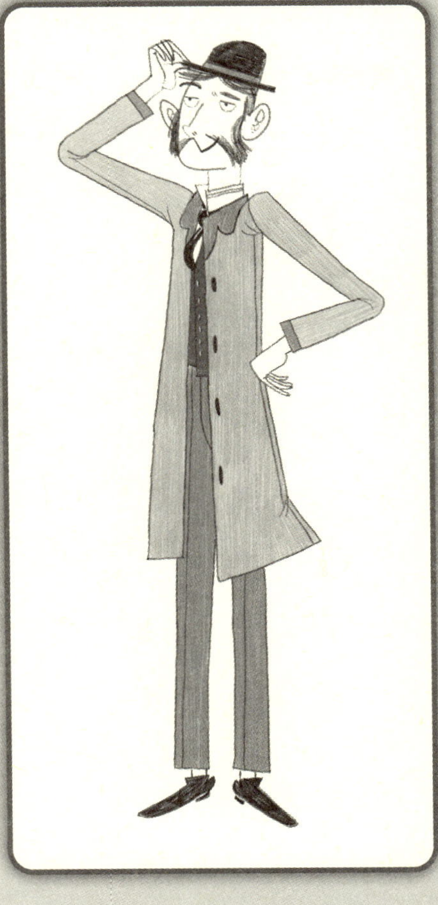

inspect - To look at something closely to find out more about it.

Sherlock touched the man's skin. He smelt his face. He felt his clothes and even checked the size and shape of his shoes.

Finally, he stood up.

'You can take the body away now,' he said.

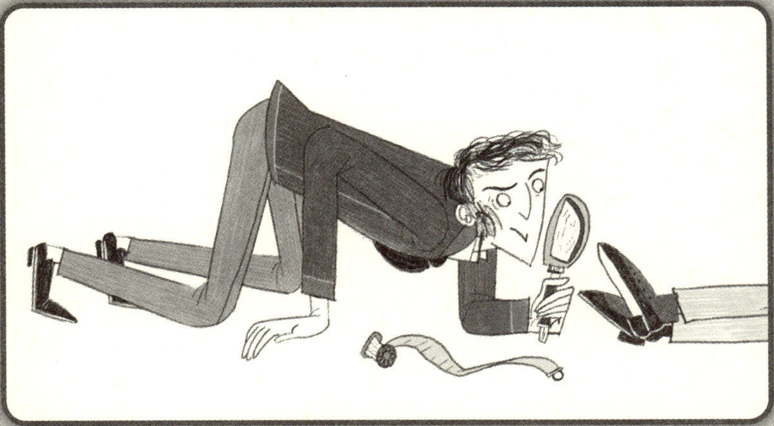

Policemen came into the room to take the body away. As they lifted the body, a ring fell onto the floor.

'Look!' shouted Gregson. 'A woman's ring! It is a clue!'

'Perhaps a woman killed the man!' said Lestrade.

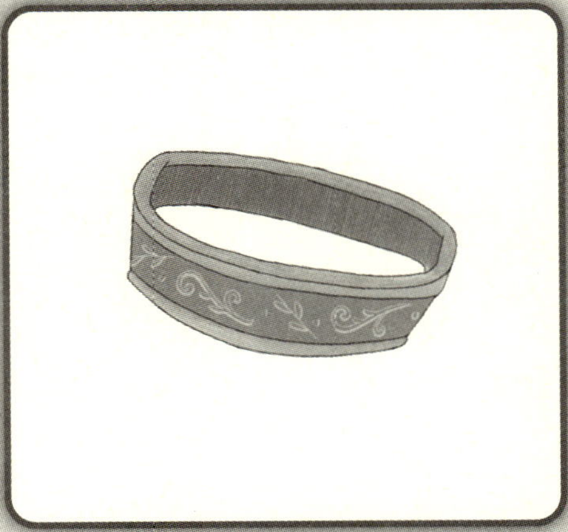

Sherlock did not agree. He asked to see everything that had been found in the man's pockets.

Gregson showed him a business card. The name on the card read: *Enoch J Drebber.* We thought that must be the man's name.

There was also a note from someone called Mr Stangerson.

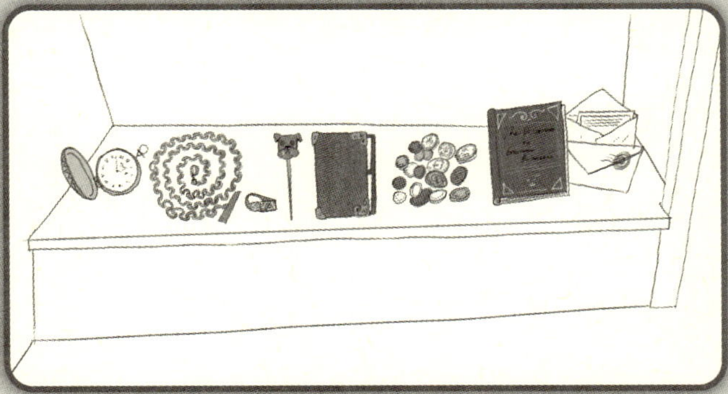

Chapter 7

'I have found something too,'

said Lestrade proudly.

He lit a match and showed us to

a dark corner of the room.

The word 'Rache' was written

on the wall.

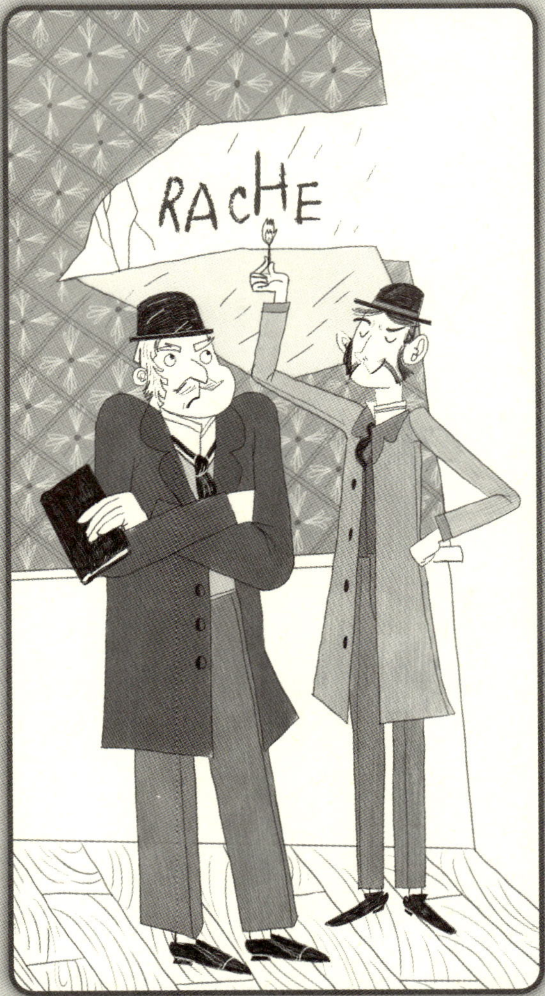
RACHE

'This is another clue,' said Lestrade. 'The **victim** wrote the name of his killer before he died. The murderer is a woman called Rachel!'

Sherlock shook his head. 'No, I don't think so.'

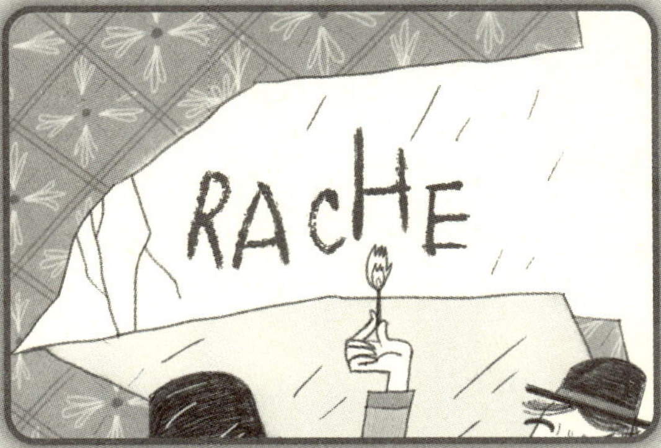

victim - *A person who has been hurt or killed.*

Sherlock asked if he could look around the room. Lestrade agreed.

Sherlock measured several things in the room. He took a **sample** of dust and dirt from the floor to test for clues.

Sherlock looked at his notes, thinking.

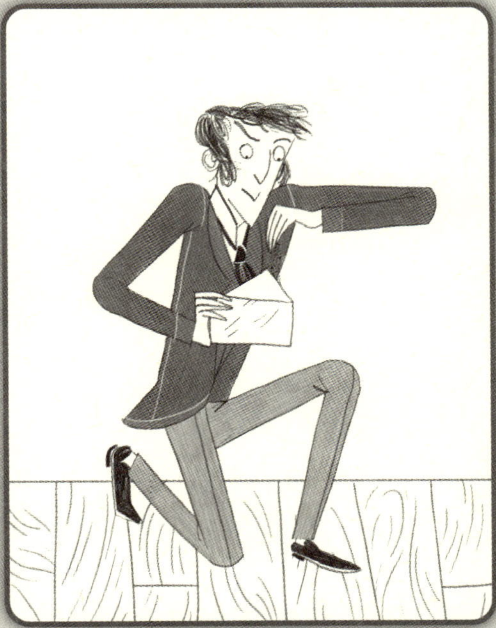

sample – A small amount of something that is tested to show what it is like.

'The murderer is six feet tall, has small feet and smokes cigars,' said Sherlock at last. 'He came here in a cab and killed his victim with **poison**. "Rache" is the German word for "**revenge**".'

The detectives stared at Sherlock in amazement.

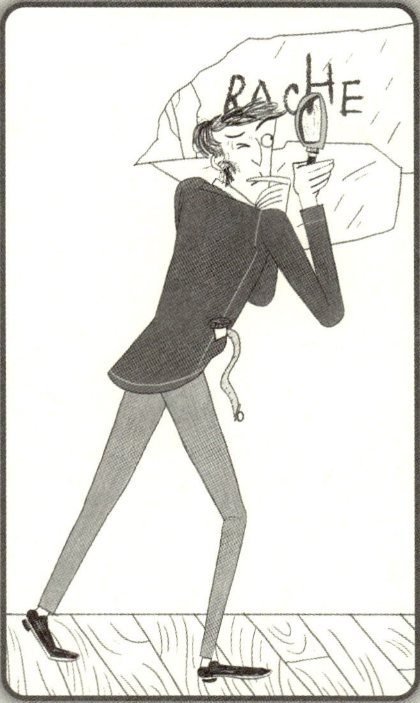

poison - *Something that a person can eat or drink that can make them ill or kill them.*

revenge - *The act of hurting or punishing someone because they have hurt you.*

Chapter 8

Sherlock told Lestrade that he wanted to speak to the policeman who had first discovered the body. His name was Constable Rance.

We got in a hansom cab to go to meet him.

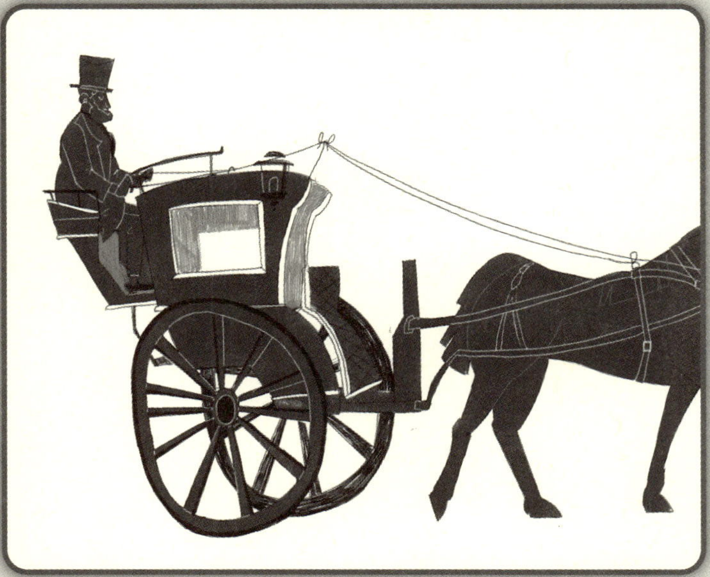

On the way, I asked Sherlock about his ***deductions****.*

'I saw ***tracks*** *on the road. A cab stopped right outside the house. There were footprints on the path that did not match the footprints of any of the policemen. The cab and the footprints must belong to the murderer,' said Sherlock.*

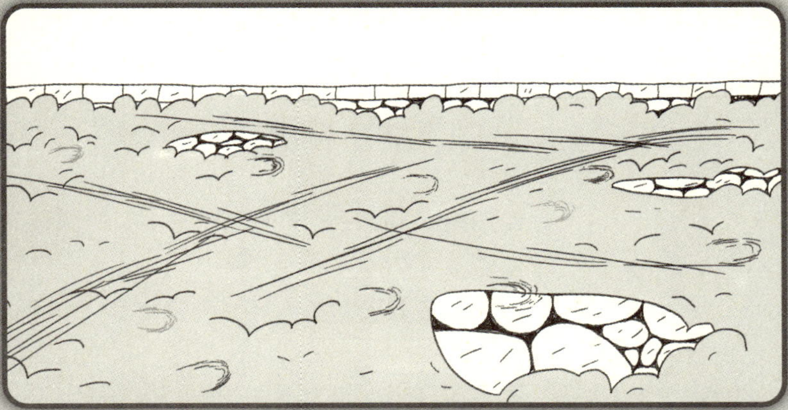

deductions - *Thoughts about what has happened, based on clues.*

tracks - *Marks made on the ground by someone or something.*

'But why did you say the murderer is tall?' I asked.

'Because he has long legs. I know this because I measured the distance between each of his footprints,' said Sherlock.

'And the cigar?' I asked.

'Simple!' said Sherlock. 'I found **ash** on the floor.'

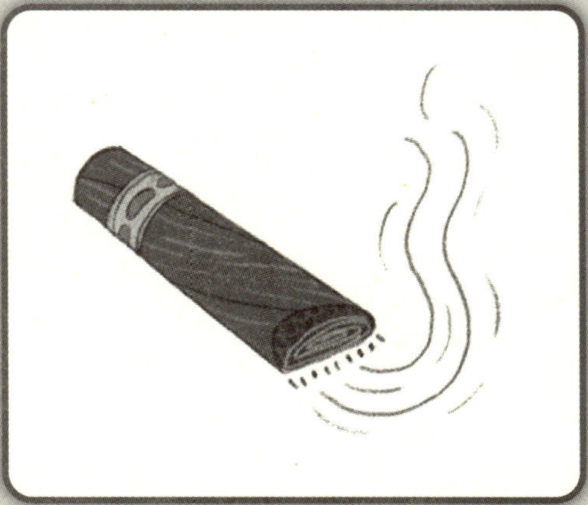

ash - Dust made from something that has been burnt.

I was amazed by Sherlock. He was by far the cleverest man I had ever met. He had discovered great clues and made super deductions. What a brilliant man!

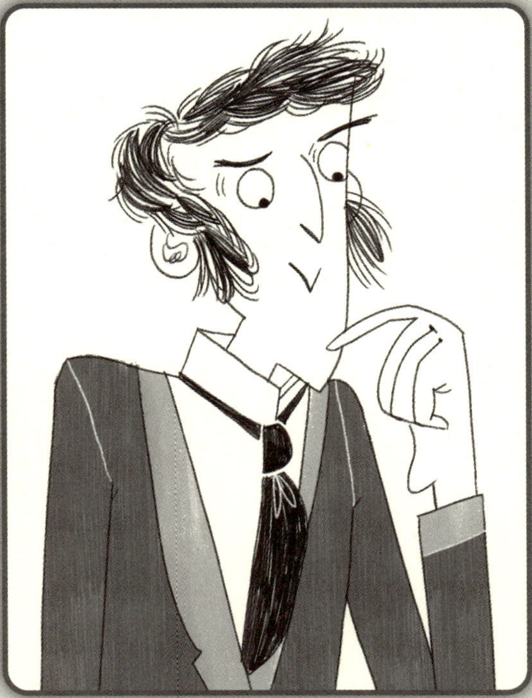

Chapter 9

Soon, we arrived at Rance's house. He was fast asleep when we knocked on his door, but the knock woke him up.

Finally, he opened the door. He was not happy to see Sherlock.

'I've told the detectives everything I know already!' he said.

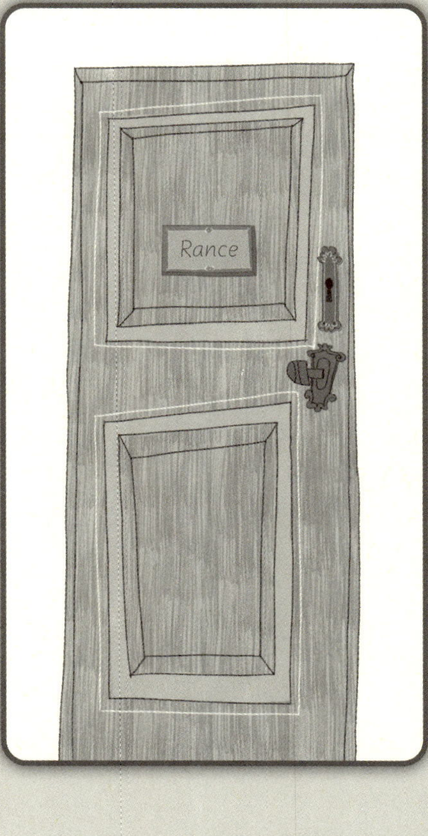
Rance

Sherlock reached into his pocket for a gold coin. When Rance saw the coin, he changed his mind.

'Perhaps I could tell my story again,' he said.

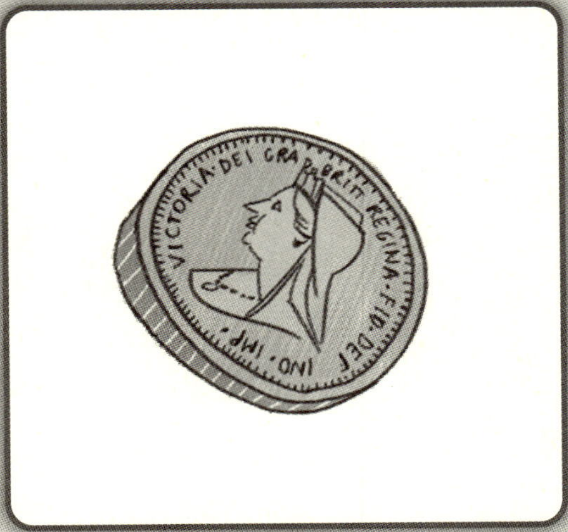
VICTORIA·DEI GRA·BRITT
REGINA·FID·DEF
IND·IMP·

Rance **explained** that he had walked past the old house in Lauriston Gardens.

'The house is usually dark and empty,' said Rance. 'But early this morning, there was a light on. So I looked through the window.'

'What did you see?' asked Sherlock.

'I saw a body on the floor,' said Rance.

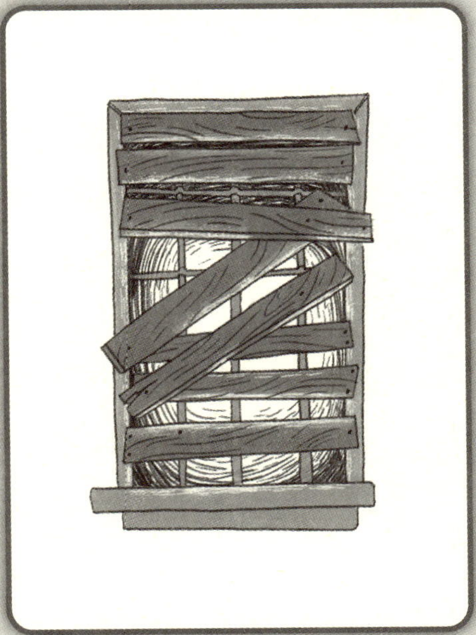

explained - Gave details about something to make it easier to understand.

'Did you see anyone else?'

asked Sherlock.

'Just an old man waiting in the street,'

said Rance.

'What did he look like?'

asked Sherlock.

'He was tall and wore a brown coat,'

said Rance.

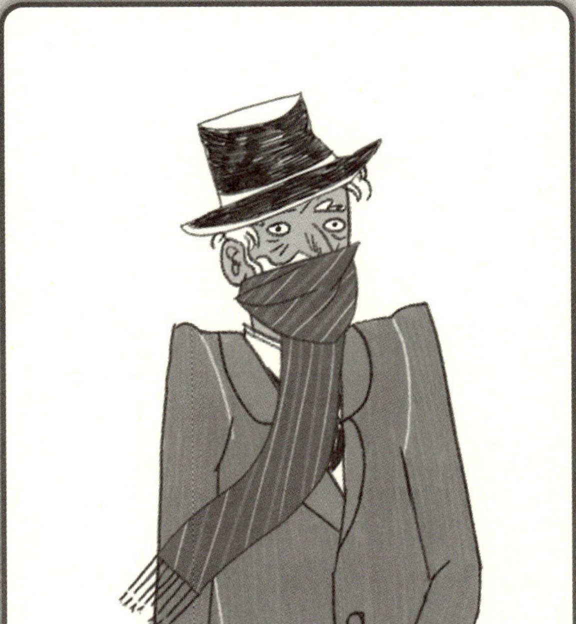

When we got back in the cab, Sherlock was upset.

'What is wrong?' I asked.

'The old man that Rance saw was the murderer!' he said. 'He must have come back to get the ring.'

I was shocked.

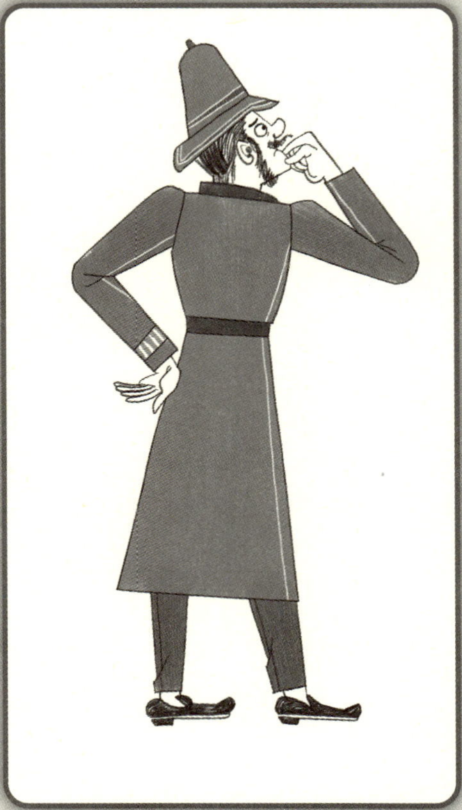

Chapter 10

A few days later, I was relaxing at home.

I decided to read the newspaper with a cup of tea.

As I was reading, I saw a **notice** *that surprised me.*

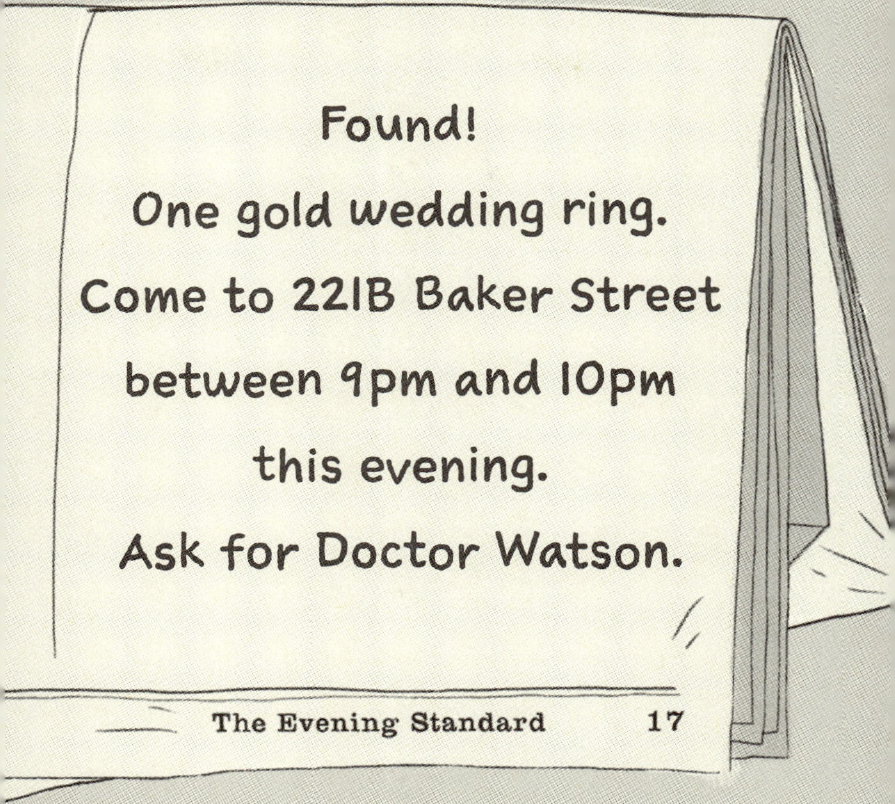

Found!

One gold wedding ring.

Come to 221B Baker Street between 9pm and 10pm this evening.

Ask for Doctor Watson.

The Evening Standard 17

notice - *A piece of information written in a place where everyone can read it.*

Sherlock had put an advert in all of the London newspapers.

He knew the murderer wanted the ring. Now he could come and collect it, and we could catch him!

It was a very clever plan.

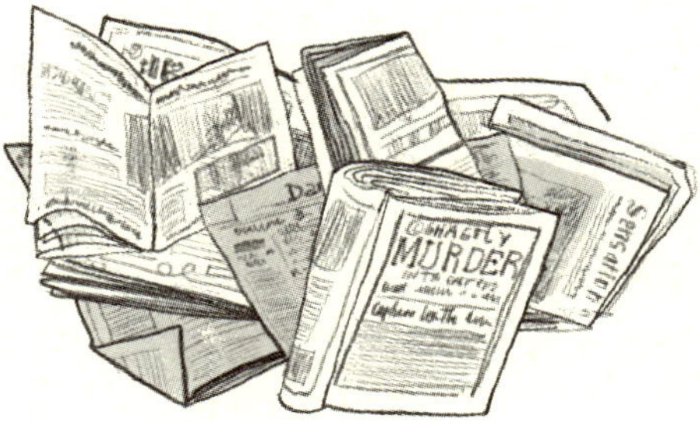
MURDER

That night, an old woman knocked on the door. She said that her daughter had lost the ring.

Sherlock gave her an old gold ring. It was not the ring that had dropped from the body.

The old woman said thank you and left.

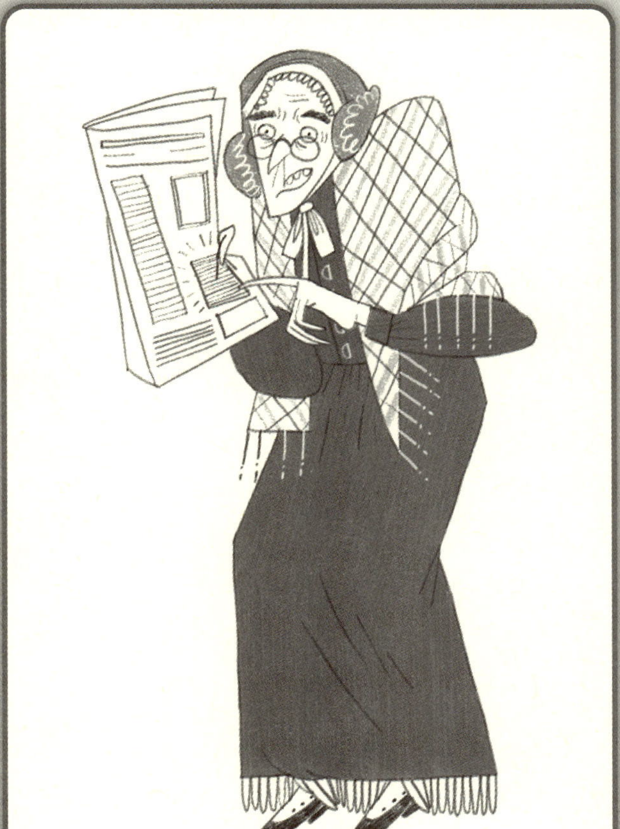

'She might be the murderer in **disguise**!' he said.

Sherlock waited a moment, then he followed the woman.

I waited for Sherlock for a long time. Suddenly the door swung open.

Sherlock was stood in the doorway. He looked tired and disappointed.

'The woman got away!' he said.

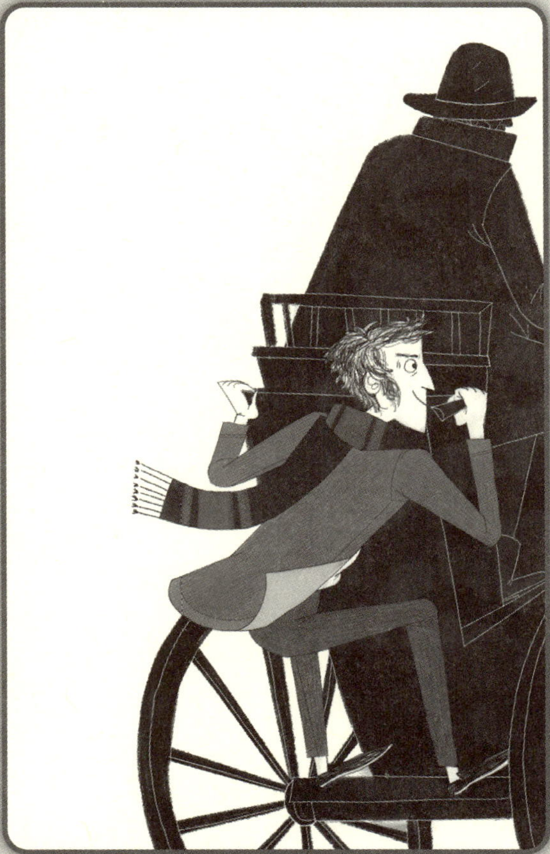

disguise - A costume that changes how you look so that you can't be recognised.

Chapter 11

The next morning, Sherlock and I heard a knock on the door.

Sherlock answered it.

It was Gregson and Lestrade. They had some more news.

'Someone else has been killed!' said Lestrade. 'Do you remember Mr Stangerson? He wrote the note we found in the dead man's pocket.'

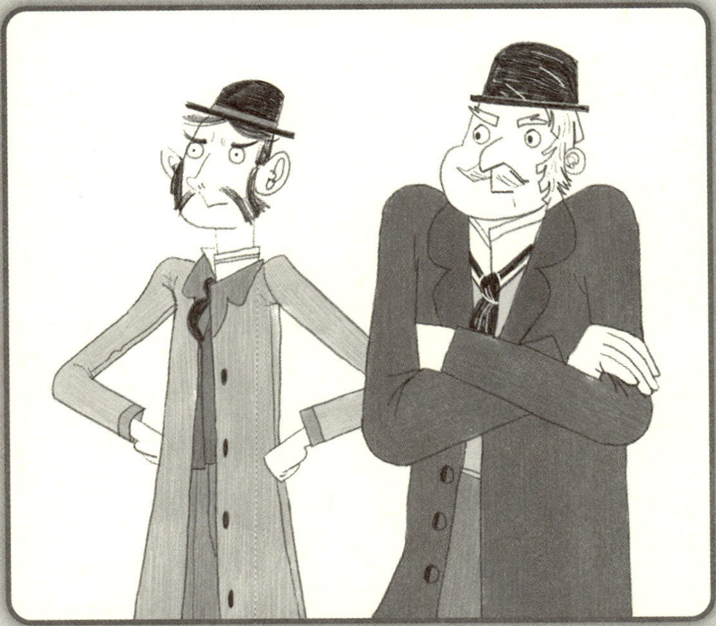

We were all shocked that someone else had been killed.

Lestrade told us what he knew about Mr Stangerson's death. He said he had been stabbed in his hotel room.

They had found two **pills** by his bed – a white one and a red one.

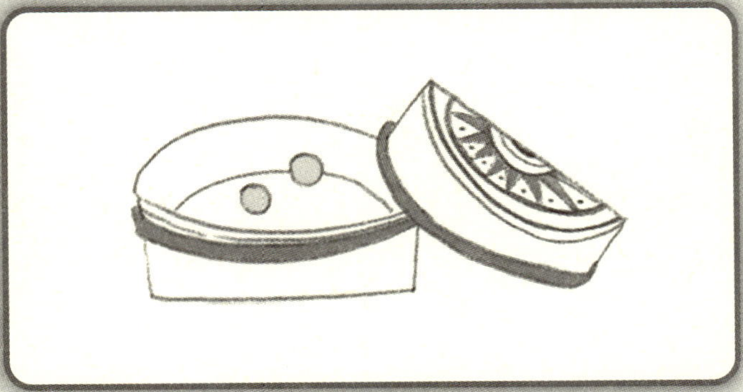

pills - *Small tablets made of powder. They are usually medicine.*

Sherlock jumped up. 'That's it!' he said. 'I have solved the crime! Lestrade, do you have those pills with you?'

Lestrade took a small tin out of his bag and gave it to Sherlock.

Sherlock took the tin with the pills inside. He then began mixing some **chemicals** together.

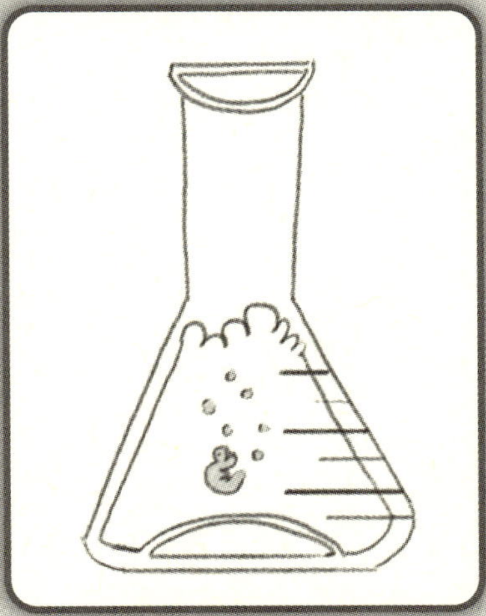

chemicals - *Substances, such as liquids, powders and gases, which are used in science experiments.*

Sherlock put each of the pills into different bottles. He then poured the mixed chemicals into the bottles, on top of the pills.

After a moment, the chemicals in one of the bottles turned red. The other stayed **clear**.

'Gentlemen, one of these little pills is poison,' said Sherlock. 'The other is harmless.'

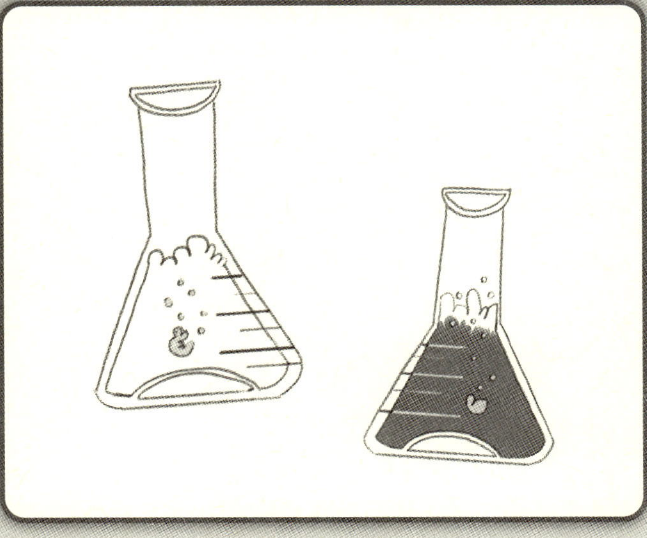

clear - *See-through.*

'What does this all mean?' I asked. 'Why did Mr Stangerson have the pills? Why was he stabbed?'

It was all very confusing.

Lestrade and Gregson did not understand either. They said they needed to go back to the police station.

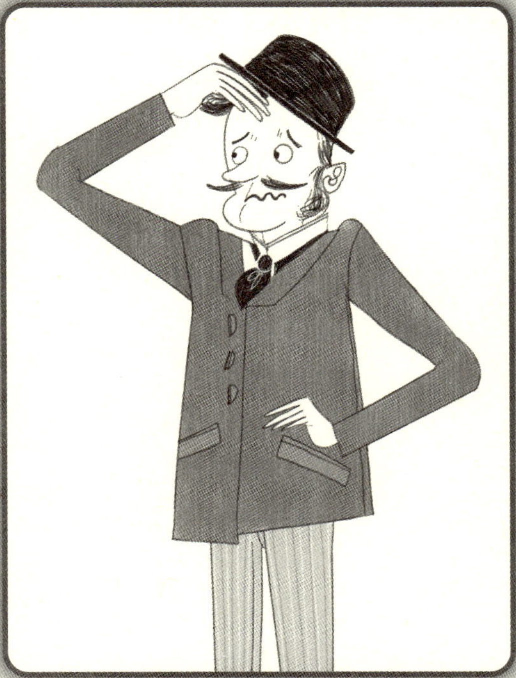

Chapter 12

We stopped a hansom cab and asked to go to the police station.

The driver was tall and wore a brown coat. As soon as Sherlock saw him, he put him in **handcuffs**.

'What are you doing?' asked the driver.

'Making sure you don't run away,' said Sherlock. 'You are a murderer!'

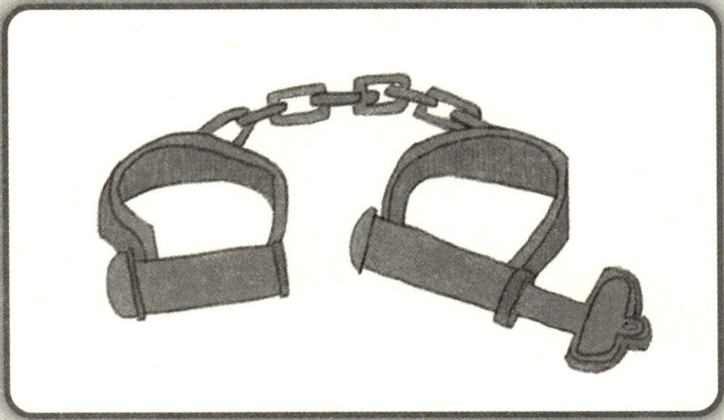

handcuffs - Two metal rings that are joined together. They can be locked around someone's wrists to stop them escaping.

The cab driver tried to escape but Gregson and Lestrade jumped on him. They put him in the back of the cab. I drove the cab to the police station.

At the police station, Sherlock spoke to the cab driver. 'Did you kill Mr Drebber and Mr Stangerson?' he asked.

'I did,' **confessed** the cab driver.

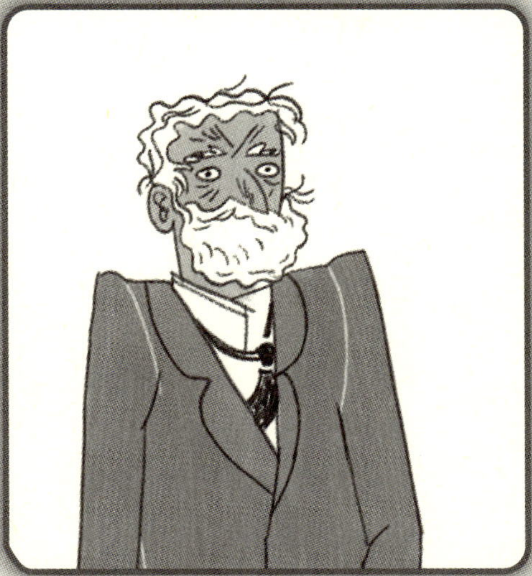

confessed - Admitted to a bad mistake or crime.

Chapter 13

Sherlock explained that the cab driver was the old man who had been seen near the house in Lauriston Gardens. His name was Mr Hope.

'I will tell you everything,' said Mr Hope. 'But I need to do it quickly. I am very ill. I have a serious problem with my heart.'

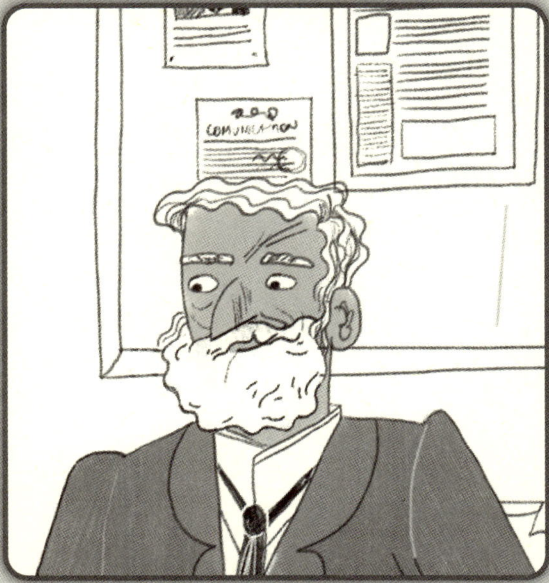

I quickly examined Mr Hope.

'This man might die very soon,' I said. 'If we want to hear his story we need to listen to it now.'

Gregson and Lestrade agreed. We all **gathered** in a room at the police station.

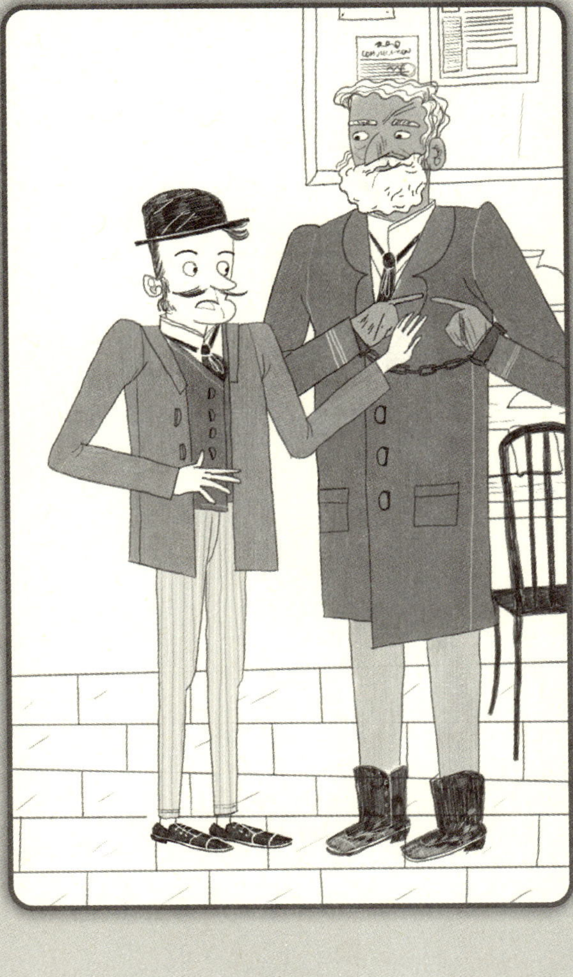

gathered - *Came together in a group.*

Mr Hope told his story.

'Twenty years ago, I visited a small town in America. I saw a lady riding a horse, but her horse was upset. I helped the lady.

'The lady's name was Lucy. I quickly fell in love with her.

'We spent almost every day together. We decided to get married.'

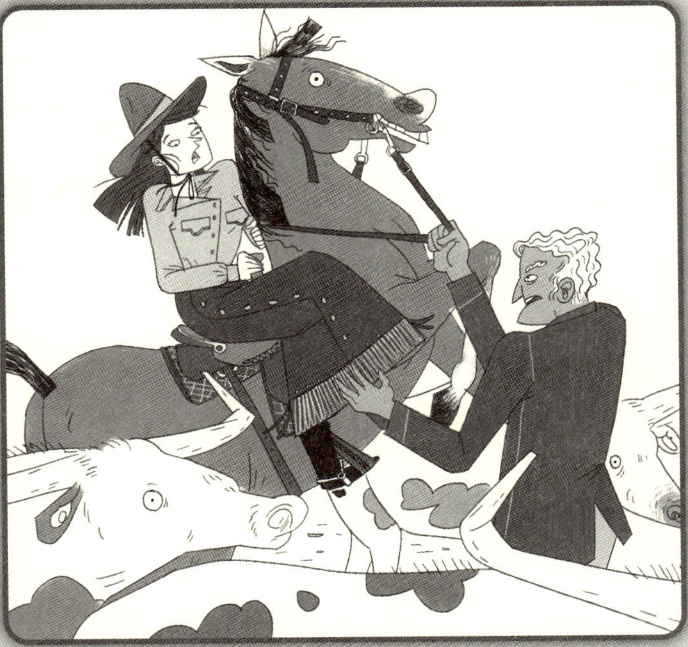

'But one day, I had to go on a **business trip** for a month. When I got back, everything had changed. Lucy was upset,' said Mr Hope.

He paused, then said, 'Lucy said she couldn't marry me. Her father had been **threatened** and he told her that she must marry a man from her town. She had to choose between Mr Drebber and Mr Stangerson.'

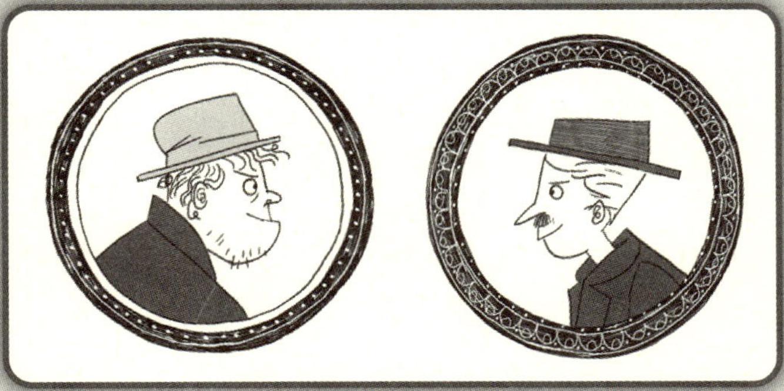

business trip - A journey made for work.

threatened - Made to feel unsafe.

Chapter 14

Mr Hope explained that Lucy did not want to marry either of the men. She wanted to marry Mr Hope.

'One night, I helped Lucy to escape. I helped Lucy's father escape too,' said Mr Hope.

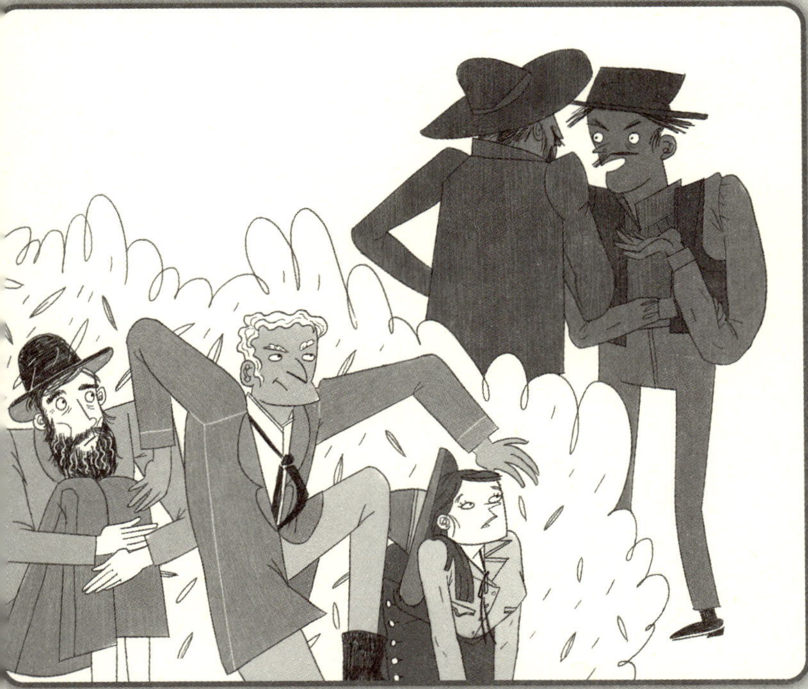

'We travelled for many days. But soon we ran out of food,' said Mr Hope. 'I built a shelter for Lucy and her father. I told them to stay there while I went to get some food. But when I got back, Lucy had disappeared and her father was dead!'

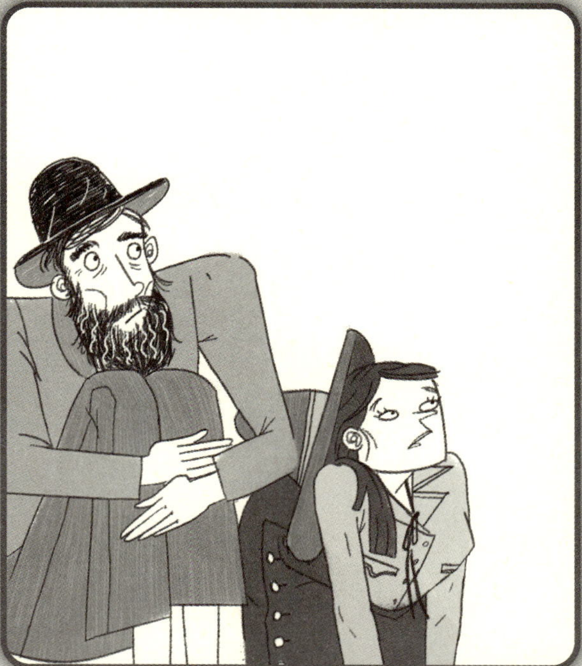

Mr Hope continued his story with tears in his eyes.

'I soon found out that Lucy had been taken back to the small town. She was made to marry Mr Drebber. By the time I got back, Lucy had died of a broken heart. I kept her wedding ring to remind me of her.'

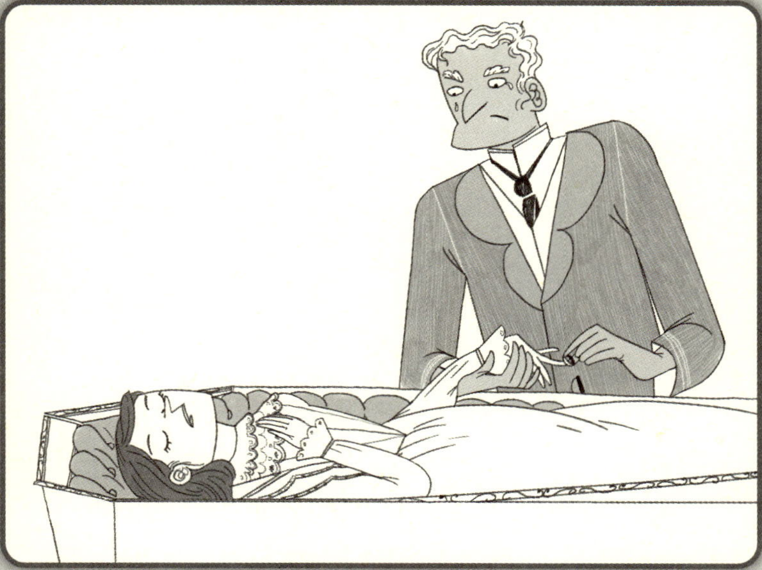

Chapter 15

'But that happened twenty years ago,' said Lestrade. 'You need to explain what has just happened.'

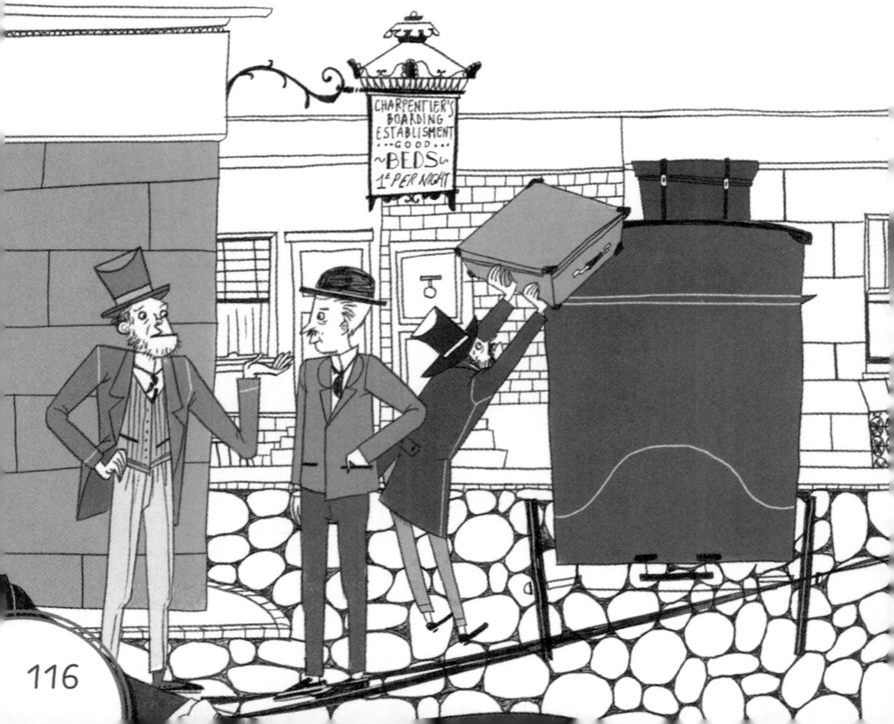

'Last month, I found out that Mr Drebber and Mr Stangerson had come to England,' said Mr Hope. 'I became a cab driver so I could follow them around London without being noticed.'

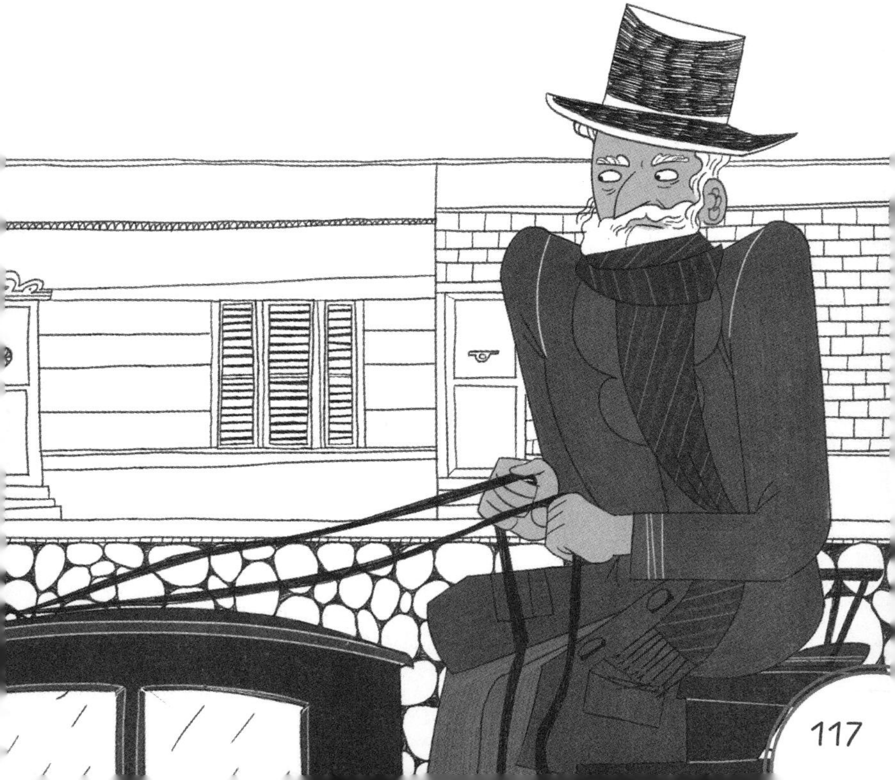

'One night, I picked up Mr Drebber in my cab,' said Mr Hope. 'I took him to the old house. I was still very angry about what had happened to Lucy. I always carried her wedding ring in my pocket.'

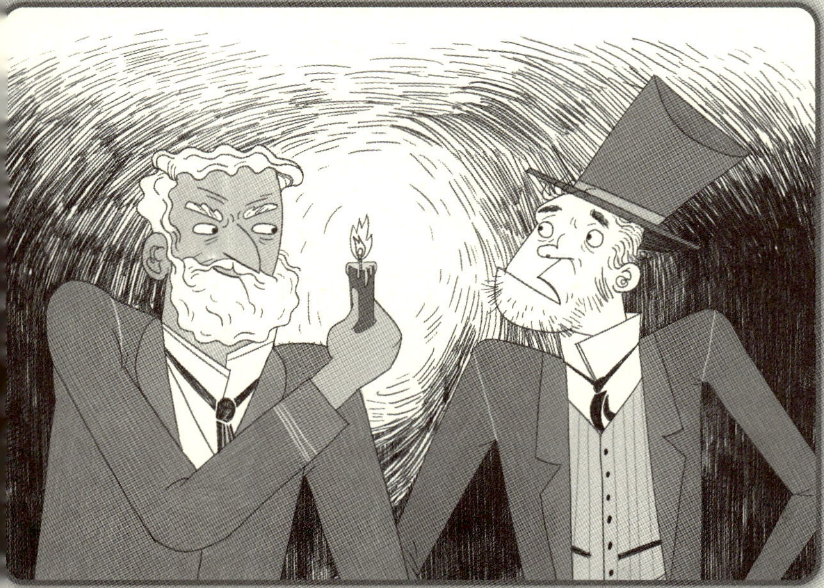

'I offered Mr Drebber two pills,' said Mr Hope. 'One pill was poisoned. The other one wasn't. Mr Drebber took the poisoned pill and died.'

'You dropped the ring in the house!' said Sherlock.

'Yes,' said Mr Hope. 'When I went to get it back, the policeman saw me.'

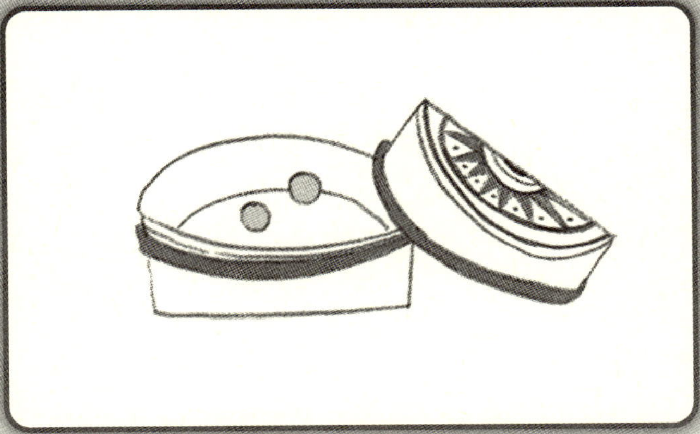

Mr Hope finished his story.

'I tried to kill Mr Stangerson with pills too. But he had a knife, so I stabbed him instead,' he said.

We all felt sorry for Mr Hope, but murder was a serious crime.

'You should not have killed Mr Drebber and Mr Stangerson,' said Sherlock.

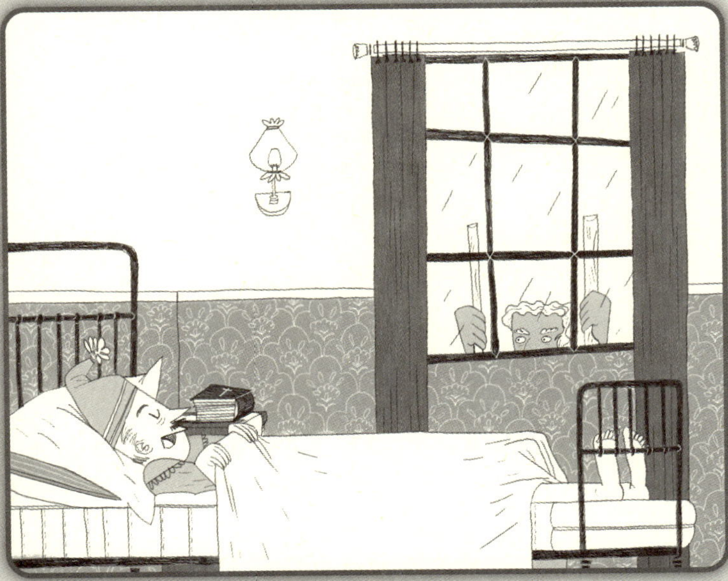

Chapter 16

Lestrade kept Mr Hope at the police station. A few days later, Mr Hope died. His heart was broken, like Lucy's.

That afternoon, Sherlock and I sat in our living room. We were talking about the case that Sherlock had just solved.

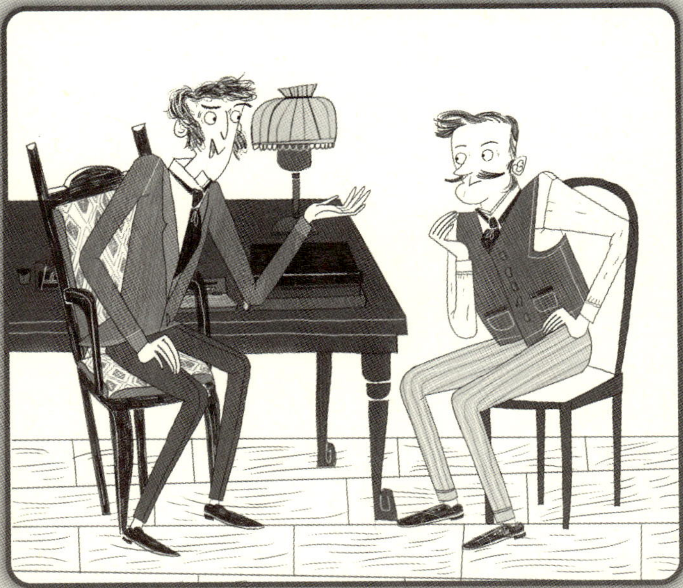

'How did you work it all out?'

I asked.

'I saw cab tracks, so I knew a cab had driven Mr Drebber to the house. I **deduced** that the cab driver was the killer,' explained Sherlock. 'Then Rance saw an old man by the house. I **deduced** that the old man was the cab driver.'

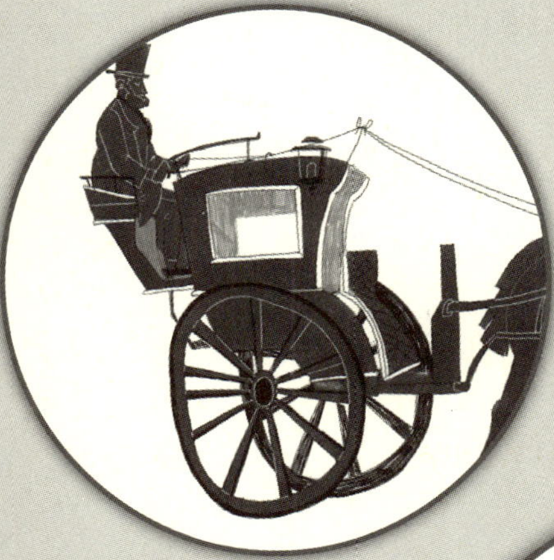

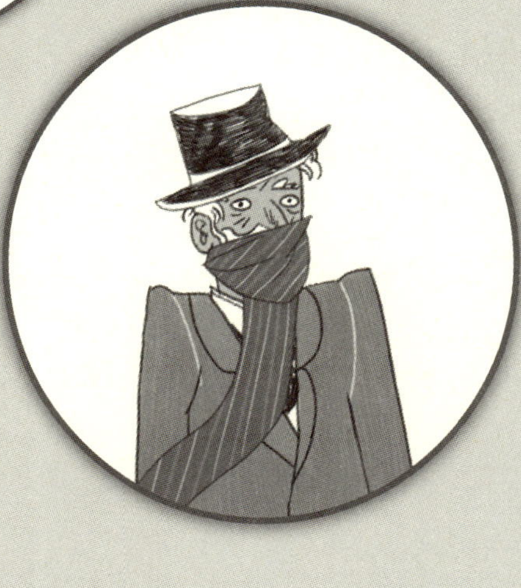

deduced - *Decided that something is true after thinking about all the clues.*

'I smelled chemicals on Mr Drebber. I deduced he was killed by poison,' explained Sherlock. 'Also, a wedding ring was dropped on the floor and the German word for "revenge" was written on the wall. I deduced it was a crime about love.'

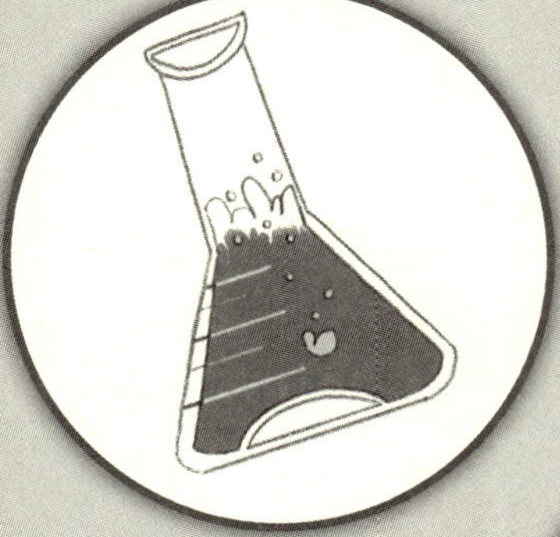

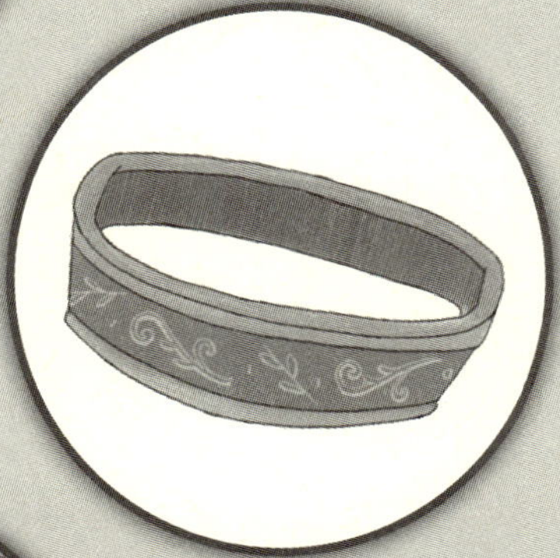

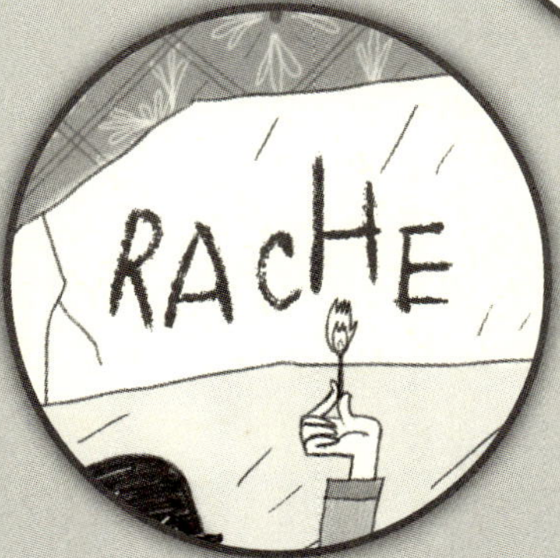
RACHE

'Finally,' said Sherlock, 'when Mr Stangerson was killed, Lestrade found the pills. As soon as I saw the pills, I knew what had happened.'

It seemed so simple when Sherlock explained it.

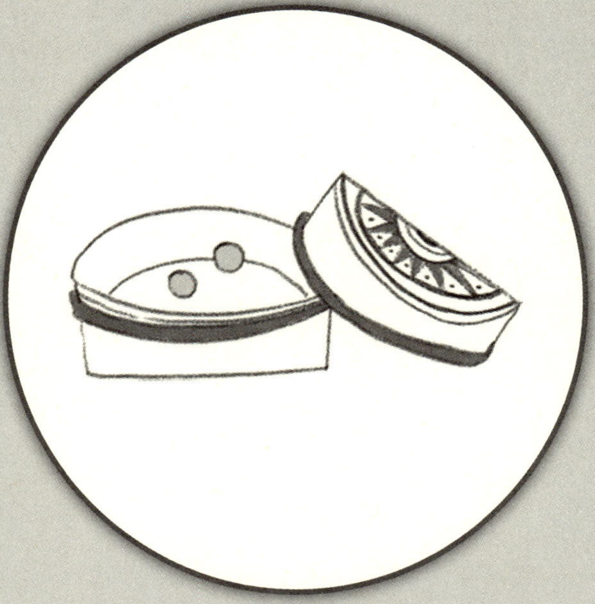

I wondered what would happen next.

One thing I could be sure of was that my life would never be dull with Sherlock Holmes around!

The End.

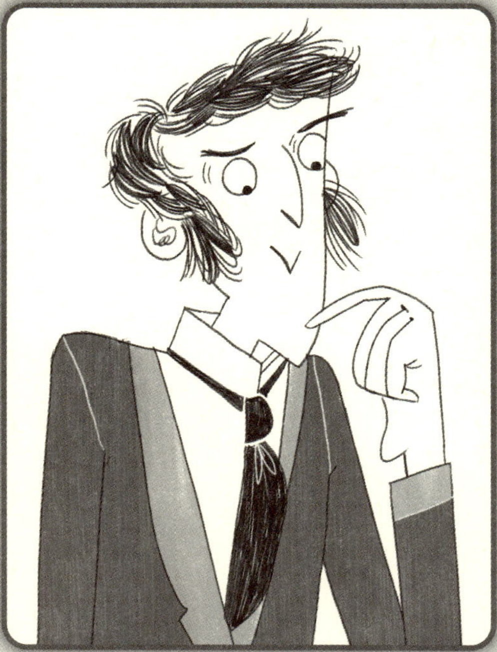

Sherlock Holmes

Sherlock Holmes is a very famous detective. He has solved hundreds of crimes! He can always find clues that many people can't.

He enjoys playing the violin and keeps bees in his free time.

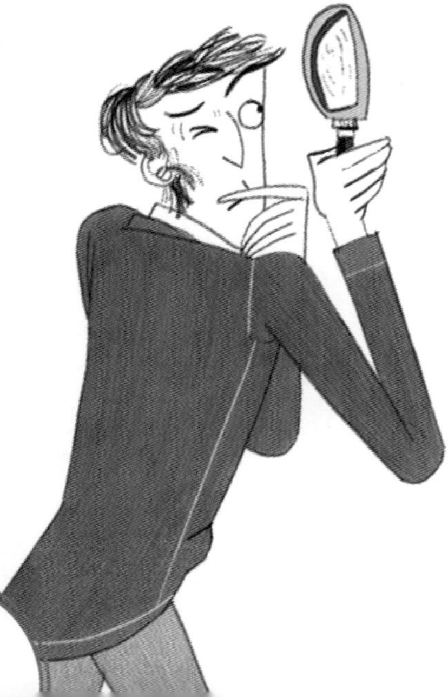

Doctor John Watson

Doctor John Watson was hurt when he was a doctor in the army. He came back to London and moved in with Sherlock Holmes. He soon learnt that Sherlock solved crimes and began to write about them.

Doctor Watson works as a doctor, and helps Sherlock to solve crimes in his free time.

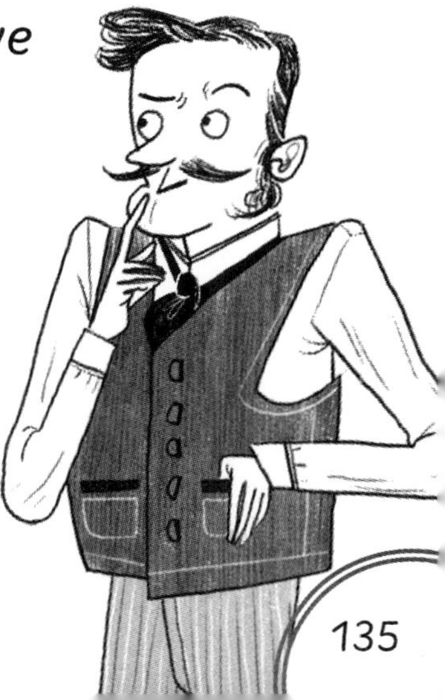

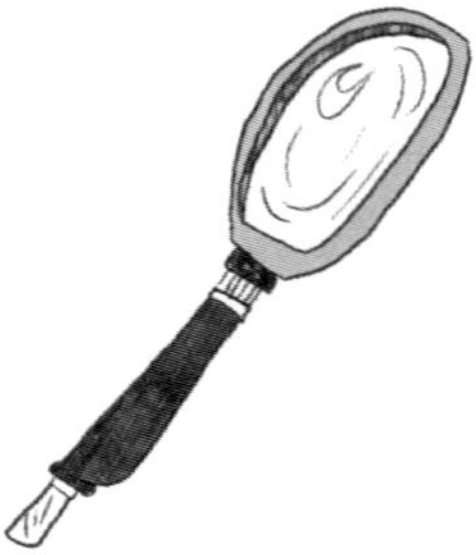